Mindful Eating

Eat Mindfully for Better Emotional and Physical Health

RON KNESS

ISBN-13: 978-1975988937
ISBN-10: 1975988930

Contents

Disclaimer

We hope you enjoy reading our report, however we do suggest you read our disclaimer. All the material written in this document is provided for informational purposes only and is general in nature.

Every person is a unique individual and what has worked for some or even many, may not work for you. Any information perceived as advice by must be considered in light of your own particular set of circumstances.

The author or person sharing this information does not assume any responsibility for the accuracy or outcome of your use of the content.

Every attempt has been made to provide well researched and up to date content at the time of writing. Now all the legalities have been taken care of, please enjoy the content.

CAUTION: See your healthcare professional before starting any diet, health or exercise program!

Introduction: What is Mindful Eating?

The word "mindfulness" is misunderstood by some people. It is not a word commonly used in everyday conversations, so it's understandable if you may not be entirely sure about what it means. Mindfulness is simply...

"The quality or state of being conscious or aware of something."

How many times have you been in a rush when eating, and you just scarfed your food down in a hurry? Have you ever woken up late, rushed around to get ready for work, flying out of the house in a hurry and pulling into a fast food drive-through to grab your breakfast because it was quicker than preparing one at home? Unfortunately, these things happen.

We say unfortunately because this is not a very mindful way to eat.

You are not being conscious or aware of how you are eating, what you are eating, and your mindset and emotions as you eat. You are eating while you are stressed out. Stress leads to inflammation and inflammation can cause your digestive system to work improperly. So, when you are stressed out as you are eating, even if you eat healthy food, your body does not process it properly.

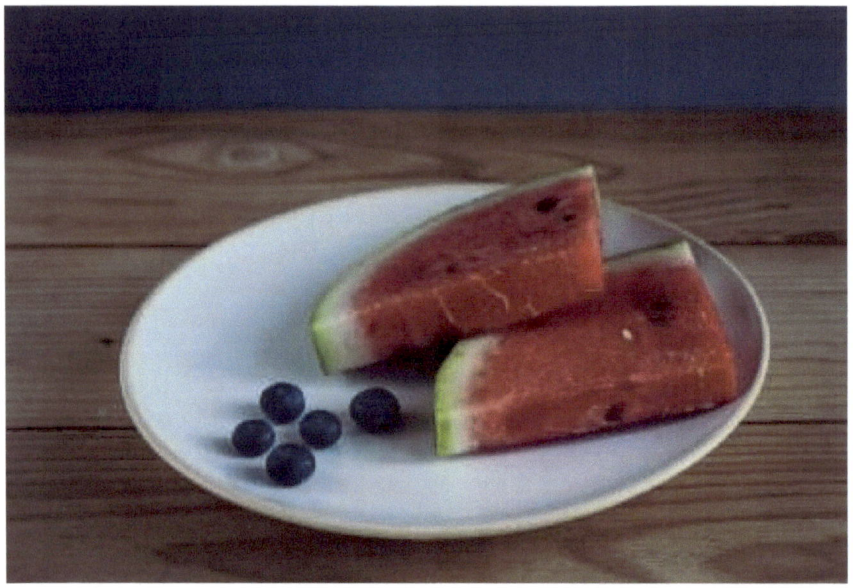

The Dangers of Mindless Eating

Research tells us that when you do not consciously pay attention to your entire eating experience, and eat "in the moment", you promote unhealthy conditions such as:

- Becoming overweight
- Obesity
- Cancer
- Diabetes
- Heart disease

When you don't take a conscious approach to nutrition, what you eat and how you eat, and the environment you are eating in, you also raise your risk of developing neurological disorders and health problems from brain fog to Parkinson's disease, and memory loss to Alzheimer's.

That's why it is so important to understand how to eat with mindfulness.

That is exactly what this report is going to help you do. In it, you will learn just exactly why junk food can be so incredibly addictive. You may have tried to put down certain foods you know are unhealthy, but found it nearly impossible to do so. Don't beat yourself up, this happens because of the intentional way food manufacturers "build" unhealthy food. They want you to be addicted to their products, and they don't really care that their food is costing you your mental and physical health.

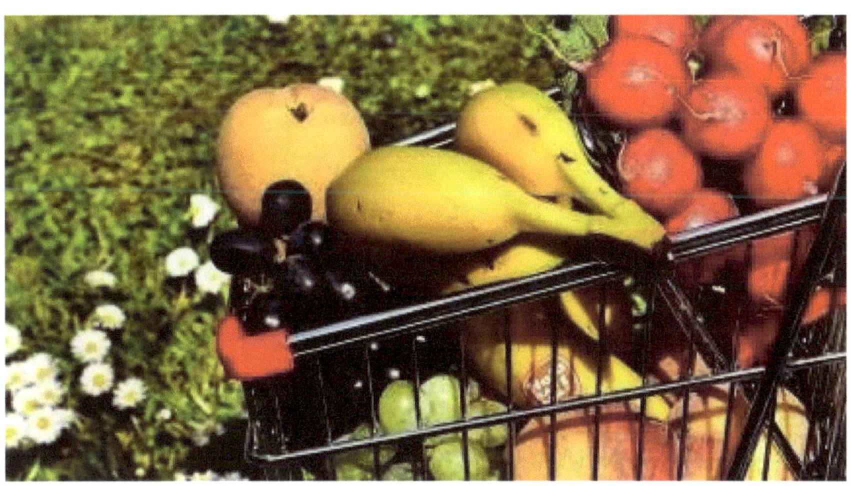

You will also discover the psychological side of overeating and food addiction. You may have a lot of good knowledge about how you should eat for health. Yet you may find yourself turning to "bad food" again and again. Why does this happen if you know what foods and eating behaviors are good and bad for your body?

In many cases, poor eating habits are tied to emotional reasons, so we will look at exactly just what emotional eating is, and how you can get a handle on it.

We will introduce you to the amazing benefits of eating mindfully, and you will find out that there are actually several different types of hunger. Determining what type of hunger you experience allows you to win and if you should be eating. You will additionally learn how to spot triggers that lead to bad eating behaviors, and the exact processes, tips and tricks that allow you to be mindful before and during your meals.

It's About Being Aware, not Perfect!

By the way, you are human, and humans make mistakes!

You need to understand that you are going to eat some less than healthy food from time to time. No problem, don't beat yourself up over this, dietary slip-ups happen. Also, it is important for you to reward yourself from time to time with a cheat meal.

For these reasons, you will discover in this mindful eating report exactly how to deal with cravings and dietary speed bumps like bacon double cheeseburgers, chocolate fudge sundaes and your favorite fast food meals.

When you become mindful, you become knowledgeable about nutrition. Being aware of what you are eating means understanding what is in the food you consume. To give you a better understanding about the nutritional principles of a healthy, mindful diet, we will look at foods like sugar, good and bad fats, salt, and we will explain smart portion control as well.

By the way, your health is not singularly created. If you are not mindful in all aspects of your life, making smart lifestyle choices, taking care of your emotions, exercising, drinking lots of water and sleeping properly, the smartest diet in the world will not give you the health rewards you're looking for. That's why we finish off this report by revealing simple mindful living and moving practices that complement mindful eating.

Let's get started creating your dream reality of emotional and physical health by looking at why so many unhealthy processed foods are so addictive, and why you overeat them rather than eating sensible amounts.

Why Junk Food is So Addictive & Why We Overeat

The first thing you need to understand about your junk food, comfort food addiction is that it is probably not an issue of self-control. Many people who want to lose weight or otherwise get in shape for some health reason are the most determined and driven individuals when it comes to their diet. Yet they still overeat. They eat bad food from time to time, or much of the time.

This doesn't seem to make sense. Yet it happens all the time. If you constantly crave sugar, salt, junk food, fast food, processed foods, TV dinners, ready-to-eat meals that you pop in the microwave and other foods you know are harmful for you, your addiction likely happens for physiological reasons that are out of your control.

In other words, **your mind responds to some unhealthy food just like an addict's brain responds to and craves cocaine, heroin or alcohol.**

Here's what happens. In short, you lose your inherent desire for a wide variety of healthy foods when you eat unhealthily most of the time. You end up programing your mind and your mouth to crave junk food.

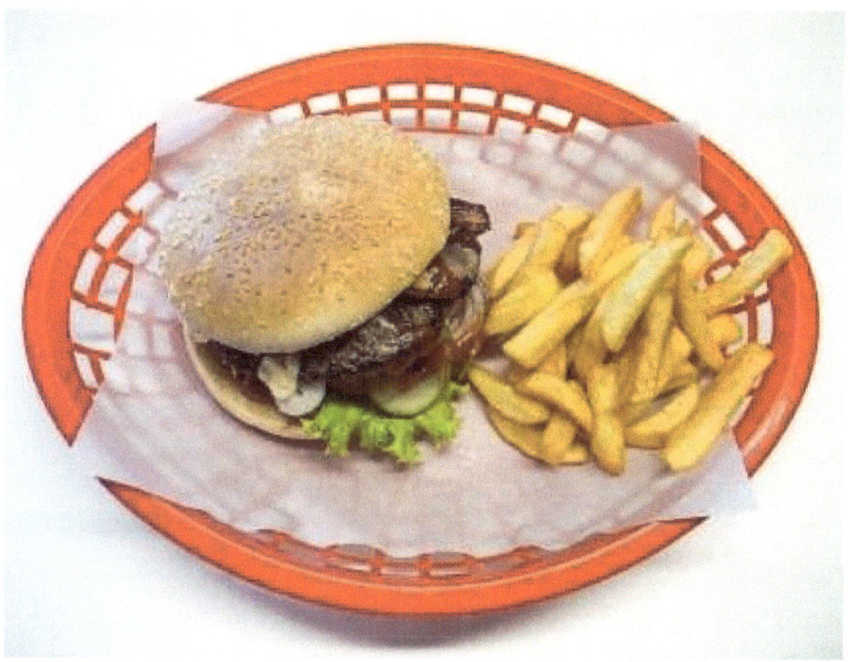

How Junk Food Affects Your Brain

When your mind and body are healthy and happy, you are hardwired to seek a variety of nutrients and foods that are good for you. This means you will crave various fruits, vegetables, nuts, berries and healthy grains – all foods that are good for you. You won't focus on eating just one type of food. This is how humans are supposed to eat.

When you overindulge on high-calorie, heavily processed foods, you cut the wires to your brain that deliver healthy eating messages. You limit the types of food you consume, and the chemicals in the unhealthy processed food you do eat, go to work programming your brain to desire them.

MSG, refined sugar, salt and other similar chemicals in most processed and fast foods go to work on the pleasure center in your brain. This means that, unfortunately, they trick your brain into thinking they are good for you. When you do things that are good for you, your brain rewards you with dopamine, serotonin and oxytocin, as well as hormones that create pleasurable feelings.

This is how you can easily and quickly become addicted to junk food... even though you know it is not good for you.

This means you start eating a limited number of foods, predominantly food that is highly processed. These types of foods have very little to no nutrition. Your mind recognizes that even though you just got finished eating, you are still nutrient-poor. It knows exactly what you need, the vitamins, good fats, enzymes, minerals and nutrients to help you exist and thrive.

Since it sees that you have not taken in any of these nutrients, it sends out a hunger signal. In this way, eating predominantly processed foods with little nutrition means you overeat daily, because your mind is telling you that it desperately needs nutrition you are not giving it.

Combined with the addictive chemicals manufacturers unintentionally and consciously put into your food to make you an unhealthy food addict, this repetitive cycle of hunger, overeating and little nutrition creates a multitude of health problems.

The takeaway is simply this ... your brain and body are set up for dietary failure if you eat unhealthy food most of the time. Your brain and body are also set up for extreme health and wellness, emotionally, physically and mentally, when you are mindfully and consciously aware of what and how you eat, and you feed your mind and body healthy, natural foods.

If this sounds like it is nearly impossible to change a chemical process that can naturally lead to poor eating habits, it isn't. In just a very short period of time, really only a few days, your brain can rewire itself so that you crave healthy food, if you eat mindfully and give your body the nutrition it needs. This means you must control your emotions, so that you don't give in to mental and psychological stressors that cause you to eat bad food in the first place.

Emotional Reasons for Junk Food Addiction & Overeating

Have you ever eaten just because you were bored? We all do. There is nothing on your 200 channels of satellite TV that interests you, all your friends are at work, you don't have a good book to read, and if it wasn't raining outside, you would go take a walk. Instead, even though you are not physically hungry, you walk into the kitchen, open your refrigerator, and fix a nice, big, unhealthy meal.

Why does this happen?

It happens because of a tight link between your emotions, your mind, your hormones, your level of fitness, and your eating behaviors. You are bored because you feel there is nothing exciting or entertaining to do. The human brain craves happiness and positive emotions, so it sends you a signal to eat. Why does it do this? This happens because your brain understands if you eat sugar, salt and other additives and preservatives in unhealthy processed food, it will trigger the release of the "feel good" chemicals we mentioned earlier.

You are bored, you eat even though you aren't hungry, you choose unhealthy food that makes you feel comfortable and happy, because the hormones that are released when this food is experienced lead to positive emotions. This kind of behavior over the long-term causes you to become physically unfit.

Studies show us that an unhealthy body promotes an unhealthy brain, and vice versa.

When you are bored and you eat improperly, you promote poor physical and mental health, even though initially, right after eating, harmful chemicals in highly processed food make you feel happy and peaceful.

By the way, boredom is not the only emotion that causes unhealthy eating habits. The phrase "emotional eating" refers to the fact that dietitians and nutritionists believe as much as 60% to 70% of all eating is driven by how you feel emotionally, not physically. Simply put, you eat to feel good, because of the process we mentioned earlier, where unhealthy chemicals and additives lead to a release of hormones that make you content.

This means if you're angry, happy, stressed, scared, frustrated, bored and have limited social input, you can overeat, and eat predominantly bad foods. *Psychology Today* magazine says the top reason for poor eating habits is unconscious eating. You have programmed yourself to be so unaware of the what, where and how of mealtime that you get stuck into the unhealthy eating cycle we mentioned earlier.

Let's take a look at some simple ways to become more aware of what your feeding habits are doing to you. These eating tips and best practices can help you avoid overeating, have proven effective for banishing unhealthy cravings, and can put you in control of your junk food addiction, rather than your highly processed and fast food favorites controlling you.

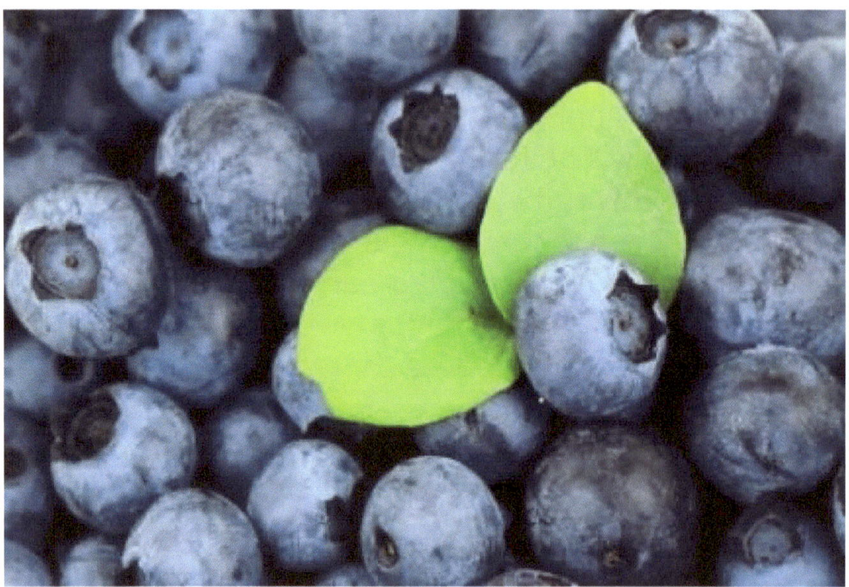

The 6 Pillars of Mindful Eating

Dr. Michelle May is the creator of the website AmIHungry.com. She offers mindful eating programs and training to help you, in her words, "Eat mindfully and live vibrantly." She has identified a simple to use 6-step process of questions you need to answer before you eat anything. This brilliantly simple, but incredibly effective way to conquer poor eating habits, has you responding honestly to the following 6 questions (The 6 Pillars of Mindful Eating) the next time you think you may be hungry for any reason.

1. Why?
2. When?
3. What?
4. How?
5. How much?
6. Where?

Let's say you are about to fix something to eat. It could be that your brain, an unhealthy food addiction, your socializing, or your emotions are driving your hunger, and not physical needs. To make sure you are going to eat for the right reasons, ask yourself...

1. **Why do I really want to eat?** Did I just get stressed out for some reason, or am I really physically hungry?

2. **When am I going to eat?** Am I eating simply because I was raised to have breakfast, lunch and dinner at a certain time? Am I about to eat simply because others around me are eating?

3. **What do I want to eat?** Am I just going to eat less than healthy food because it is nearby and handy, or do I want to eat healthy food, even if I have to take time to prepare it?

4. **How will I eat?** Am I going to eat in a hurry? Am at my car, my desk, standing, sitting, alone or with others? Am I going to eat so fast I barely taste my food, or am I going to be mindful and savor every bite?

5. **How much will I eat?** What are the factors which are driving my decision to eat a particular quantity of food? Will I eat too little and starve my body of the nutrition it needs because I think I am too fat, will I eat smart portions, or will I overeat?

6. **Where will I eat?** Do I understand is easy to my physical environment can lead to healthy or unhealthy eating behaviors?

If you are honest with yourself when answering these 6 questions, it is very difficult to eat for the wrong reasons.

By taking the time to question your behavior, you are being mindful and conscious about nutrition. Sure, you can lie to yourself when you answer these questions, but if you do, you will probably never be able to beat a junk food addiction and other unhealthy eating practices anyway.

Those are the 6 pillars of mindful eating. Ask yourself these questions before you eat, in any order or sequence, and you will eat for the right reasons and not for the wrong ones.

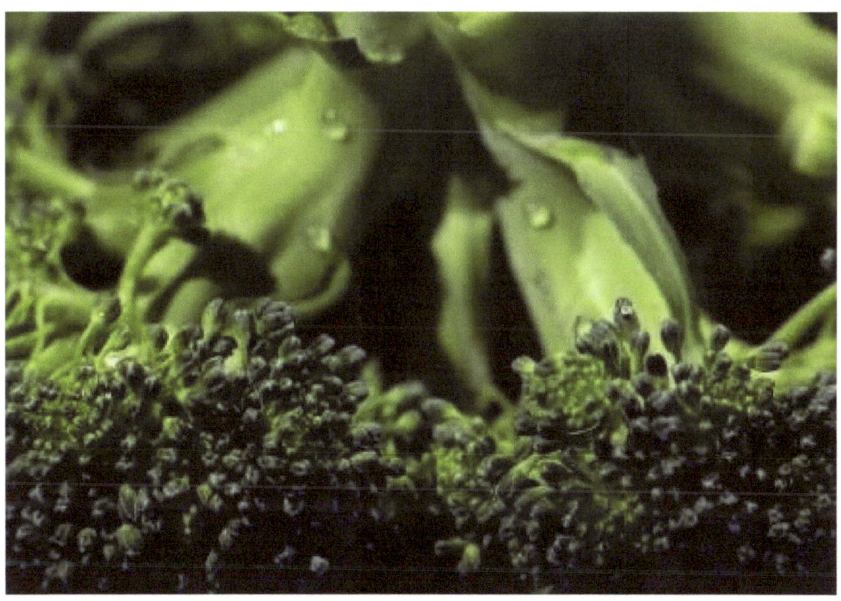

Nutritional Principles of a Healthy, Mindful Diet

The following 6 nutrition principles are straightforward and simple. They are also the solid foundation of a healthy and mindful diet.

1 – Drink water, oolong, black, green and herbal teas frequently throughout the day. Skip the soft drinks and energy drinks you know are not healthy for you.

2 – Limit or eliminate processed foods. If food comes in a carton, a box or a bag, if it has a label or a brand name, it is most likely highly processed. Stick to the outer perimeter when you shop at your favorite grocery store, because the interior aisles are where most processed food is found.

3 – Be smart with your carbs. Avoid simple carbohydrates like processed sugar, bread, pasta and baked goods. Get your carbohydrates from fruits, vegetables and whole grains.

4 – Eat lean protein at every major meal. Organic eggs, grass-fed beef and wild-caught fish are excellent sources of protein. So are broccoli, peas, artichokes, spinach, kale and Brussels sprouts.

5 – Eat 5 or 6 times a day. Plan for 3 major meals and 2 or 3 healthy snacks each day. Every time you eat, your metabolism cranks up, burning fat, calories and carbohydrates.

6 – Eat predominantly a plant-based diet, consuming foods as close to their natural state as possible. This means the bulk of a mindful diet should be fresh, whole vegetables, nuts, berries and fruits.

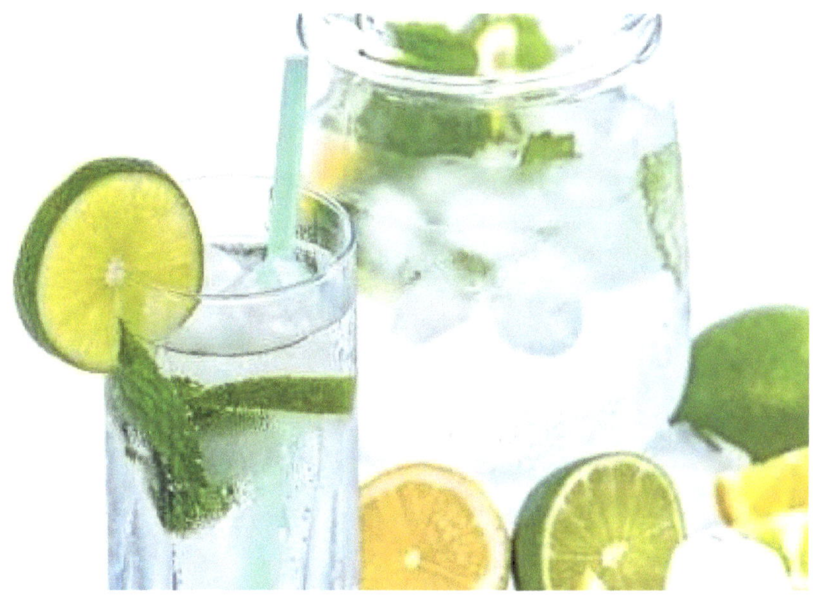

The Benefits of Mindful Eating

The Huffington Post published a really good blog post on the surprising benefits of mindful eating in 2012. They point to multiple studies that show being mindfully aware of what and how you are eating can help you...

- Lose weight
- Improve Type 2 diabetes symptoms
- Conquer eating disorders such as bulimia, anorexia and binge eating
- Reduce overeating
- Make healthy food choices, as opposed to eating unhealthy foods

- Lower your risk of developing cancer, heart disease, diabetes and brain-based disorders

When you become aware of what you are eating, it is easier to make smart food choices that are good for your health. This can lead to the above benefits, as well as literally any mental or physical health boost you are seeking. When you feed your body and mind the foods they naturally crave and need to perform at their best, that is exactly what they do.

Understanding The 7 Different Types of Hunger

Dr. Jan Chozen-Bays is the author of the book *Mindful Eating*. She helps people turn on their awareness radar, especially concerning eating habits. She has identified the following 7 types of hunger.

1. **Mouth Hunger –** Are you hungry for a certain type of food because you have been socially programmed to prefer its taste and flavor over healthier food?

2. **Eye Hunger –** This is a common reason for overeating. Your taste buds are stimulated by the sight of yummy food.

3. **Nose Hunger –** Often times, the experience you think of as taste is really the smell of food. Sometimes just smelling food that you know you enjoy eating can cause you to overeat or eat when you are not hungry.

4. **Stomach Hunger –** This is "real" hunger. Your stomach begins to rumble, and it sends messages to your brain telling you that you are hungry.

5. **Cellular Hunger** – This is another real hunger as well. It happens when your cells begin the process of signaling your brain they need certain nutrients. It is hard to detect, but it is the real reason human beings eat.

6. **Mind Hunger** – Are you anxious to eat because you just started a new fad diet? Have you been doing a lot of research into nutrition? Allowing your mind to correctly and safely drive healthy eating behaviors is important, and is the focus of this report, but there comes a time when you can overthink your eating experience.

7. **Heart Hunger** – This is emotional eating. You eat to feed or placate some emotional or spiritual need, and not because you are physically hungry.

It can be difficult to distinguish between the 7 types of hunger. However, as long as you ask yourself the questions mentioned earlier, the 6 pillars of mindful eating, you can discover which type of hunger you are trying to feed every time.

Learning to read your body's individual hunger cues is one of the key parts of mindful eating.

At first, you'll simply feel hungry and just want to eat whatever you want to eat. At this stage, it's important to regularly refer to this list and the mindful eating questions.

After a while, you might start to notice some patterns – cravings certain things at specific times of the day, or wanting unhealthy foods when you're experiencing certain states of mood.

This doesn't mean you'll necessarily be able to stop feeling that hunger, however, you will start noticing when it is true hunger and when it's emotional or boredom hunger. The more you recognize it, the more you'll train your brain to end the damaging patterns!

Discovering How Much Food You Really Need

If you live in a modern, industrialized nation, you probably eat too much. Odds are you eat too much over the course of an entire day, and you also eat too much at each meal.

The following guidelines will help you control the portions of food you eat, and lead you down to a path of total health when you consciously control the amount of food you consume. Combine these with learning as much as you can about the types of hunger explained above, and you'll have the recipe for a much more mindful diet.

- Remember, everyone is different. Don't eat a certain type or amount of food just because that is what someone else is eating.

- Chew your food slowly, take time to eat, and enjoy the experience. It takes roughly 30 minutes for your mind to know if you are full or not, so take your time and enjoy your meals.

- Pay attention to the process. Look at your food. Feel it when it enters your mouth. Savor the aroma, taste, flavor and texture. Eat one bite at a time. Be consciously aware of every step of the meal preparation and eating processes.

- If you think you are hungry, drink a glass of water and wait 10 minutes. If you still experience hunger, it may very well be that you are physically in need of food.

- Eat "real food", foods found in nature. They naturally regulate appetite, and can keep you from consuming too many calories, and the wrong types of foods.

- You should be eating at least 5 to 7 servings of fresh fruits and vegetables every day. You don't have to count calories, carbohydrates or fats with natural foods like these.

- Track what you eat. Track your health metrics as well. Doing this will help you understand exactly how much you need to eat over time, to deliver specific health results.

Being Mindful While You Eat

Remember the definition of mindfulness mentioned at the start of this report? Being mindful is "The quality or state of being conscious or aware of something." The following practices will help you be conscious, aware and mindful of every step of the eating process.

- Chew slowly. You will hear that recommendation throughout this report, since it is one of the easiest ways to be more aware at mealtime.

- Watch your posture. Slouching and laying down while eating put a great strain on your digestive system. You get the most nutrients out of the food you eat when your back and the trunk of your body, as well as your head, are perpendicular to the ground.

- "Listen" to your body. Often times you may find yourself eating just for the sake of eating. If you begin to be more aware of how you feel while you eat, you can learn when you are full, and when it is time to put your fork down.

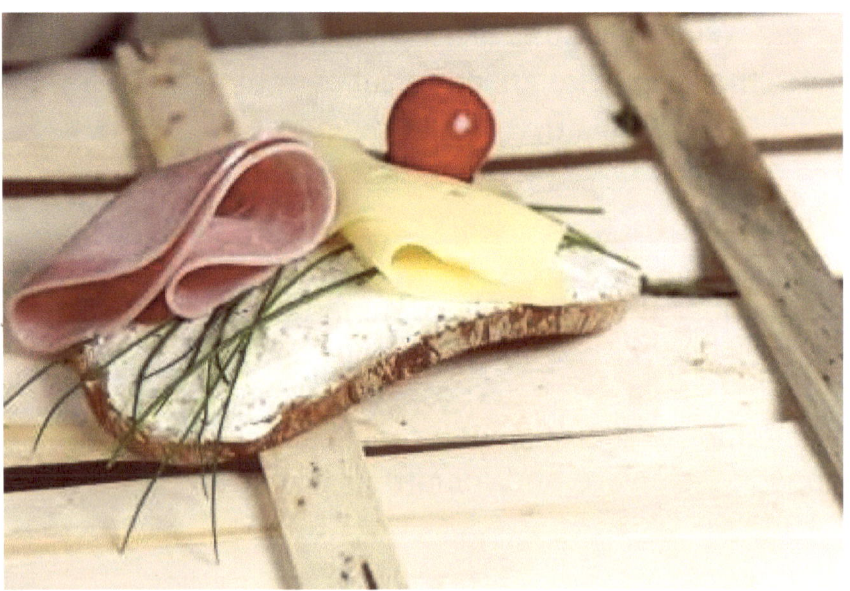

- Just eat when you eat. This means, turn off the television and your smart phone. Be aware of the eating experience, who you are eating with, where you are eating, as well as the food you are eating.

- Acknowledge your thoughts, feelings and emotions before and during mealtime. This can help you curb unhealthy emotional eating sessions.

- Give thanks. Rather than wishing you had more food, or another type of food, be thankful that you are blessed with this meal.

- Put your fork down between bites. This is an easy way to slow down the eating process.

- Sit down. Relax. Take your time. Truly enjoy the experience.

- Eat in silence if you can.

- Eat food that requires work. If you have to peel, shell or seed food, or cut it before eating it, this can make you more aware of the process.

- Consciously change what you eat from time to time. Learn to eat a rainbow of colors, enjoying fresh, natural foods of all colors.

Dealing with Withdrawal, Cravings and Slip-Ups

Earlier we talked about asking yourself 6 simple questions to determine if you really should be eating, and what you should be eating. You can ask yourself those same questions if you feel like you are about to give into unhealthy cravings. They are also applicable after the fact if you slip up and eat some unhealthy food. Ask yourself the why, where, what, when, how and how much questions in regard to your unhealthy eating speed bump.

In the beginning of adopting a mindful, healthy eating diet you are going to experience physical and mental withdrawal behaviors. Your emotions could get out of control, and you may not even recognize yourself and your behaviors. This is normal. At first, your mind and body may betray you, and you will have nearly uncontrollable desires to binge on unhealthy food.

Tell yourself that when you experience withdrawal symptoms, this is a great sign. It means you are on the path to recovering conscious and aware eating habits. Be aware that intense cravings and the occasional mistake are going to happen when you begin to consciously change your eating habits and behaviors. When you feel you are about to lose control and make a mistake regarding eating, drink a large glass of water.

Exercise has also been proven to limit stress and promote positive feelings, two things that can help you regain control when you experience withdrawal, or you begin to crave food you know is not good for you.

Sometimes, you *will* end up giving into your cravings. Is this an excuse to stop learning, to stop trying? No!

The key is not to beat yourself up about it. Accept that you caved into your cravings, enjoy the feeling of eating the food you were craving, then happily move back to enjoying the positive benefits you get out of mindful eating.

Remember, mindful eating does not need to be all or nothing.

How to Live and Move Mindfully to Complement Your Diet

Mindful eating alone will make a huge difference in the way you feel. However, your body is meant to move, and this means that you'll really feel your best – and feel more mentally able to deal with your cravings – if you exercise alongside your mindful diet.

Multiple health authorities agree just 150 minutes of moderate physical activity each week leads to health and wellness. You can break those 150 minutes down however you like, but they should be practiced in at least 5 different sessions over a minimum of 3 days. You can alternately get the same physical fitness benefits by performing 75 minutes of vigorous, intense activity.

Sit down and mindfully write out an exercise program you can live with. Be conscious of your schedule, and things that may interfere with your physical fitness program. Tweak this schedule accordingly, write it down on paper somewhere you will see it often, and stick to it.

The types of exercise you want to focus on for these 2.5 hours are aerobic, heart-pumping exercises. This means things like ballroom dancing, jogging, running, brisk walking, an intensive gardening session, swimming, playing tennis or racquetball.

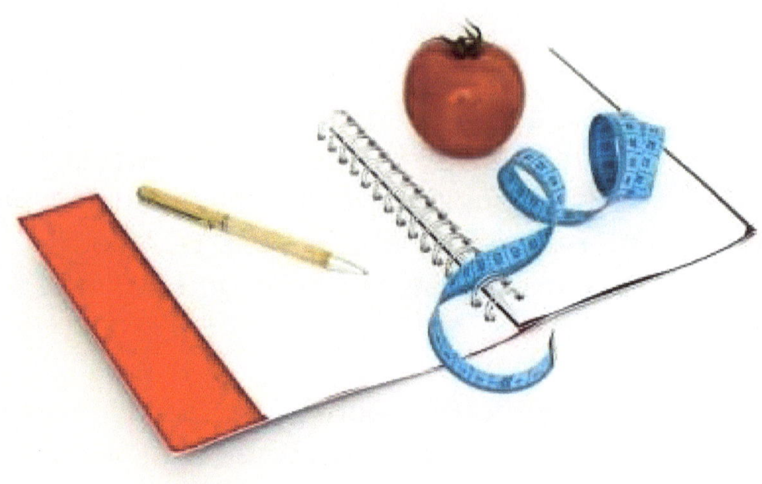

If you can talk but not sing while you are exercising, you are enjoying a moderate level of intensity. The definition of vigorous exercise is when you have to stop what you are doing to talk.

Mindful Living Tips

Mindful eating is just one part of being conscious and aware of your existence. The following mindful living tips will lead to even more emotional, physical and mental wellness.

- Walk in nature regularly, smelling, seeing, touching and hearing your surroundings.

- Meditate. Take time to breathe deeply, calm your mind, clear your thoughts and just focus on the current moment. Don't think about the future or the past, and concentrate on nothing.

- Focus on one task at a time. The myth of productivity being linked to multitasking is just that, a myth.

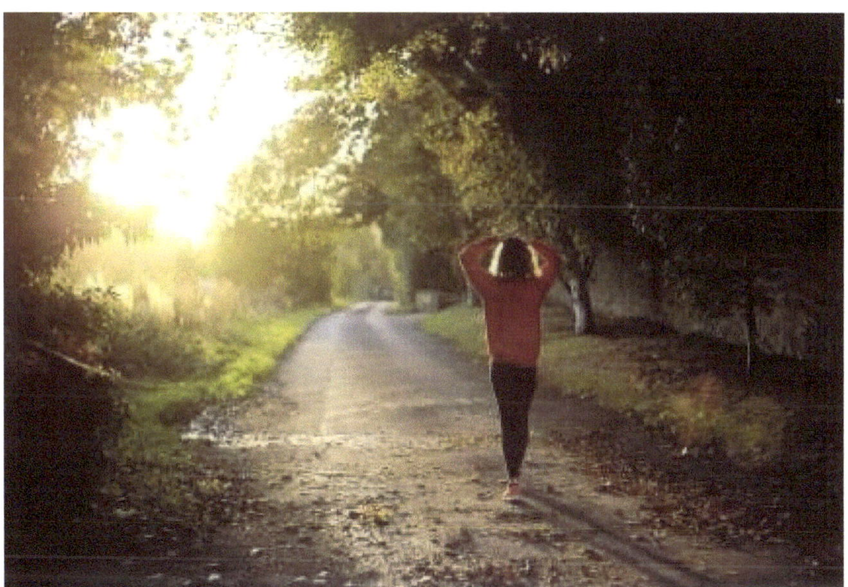

- Plan unplugging sessions every day. Detaching yourself from all consumer-electronics on a regular schedule can help you reach a mindful awareness of yourself and your existence, as opposed to your reaction to massive amounts of uncontrolled electronic sensory input.

- Appreciate yourself. Instead of knocking yourself down for perceived negative traits or characteristics, take time every day to recognize and verbally appreciate your positive attributes and skills.

- Consciously drink water throughout the day.

- Be conscious of what you put into your mind. Your mental fitness dictates your physical health, and vice versa.

- Get plenty of rest. If you are not rested upon waking, it is hard to practice mindfulness and become conscious of your life.

- Recognize failure as an event, not as who you are. If you make a mistake or fail, that is simply something that happened, and it does not become who you are.

- Simplify. Minimize. You don't own your possessions, they own you. When you have more things than you need, you are distracted and hectic, rather than being aware and focused.

Take it One Step at a Time

Remember, mindful eating is not a diet, it's a lifestyle shift. This means that you can take it gradually, one step at a time. You don't need to be perfect, and you shouldn't expect results overnight.

The good news is that the results you will see won't just be physical, they'll also be psychological and lead to a healthier, happier life.

Bonus Downloads

Register Your Mindful Eating Guide at
http://healthylifestylenewsletter.com/mindfuleating/
MindfulEatingRegistrationPage.html

and Receive the Five Bonuses Below:

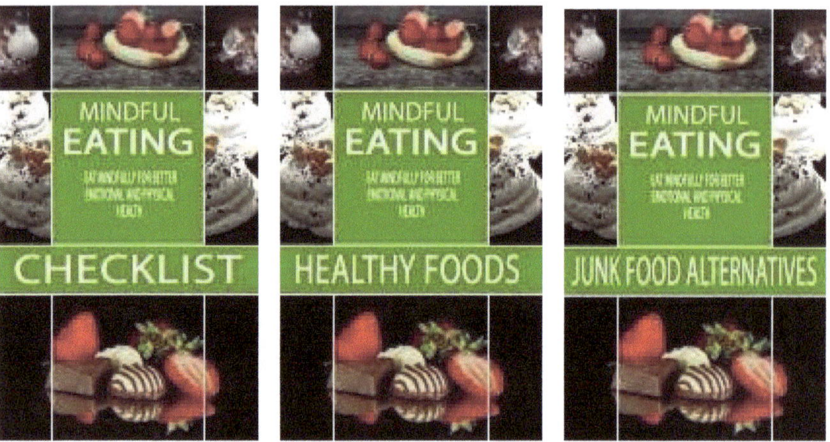

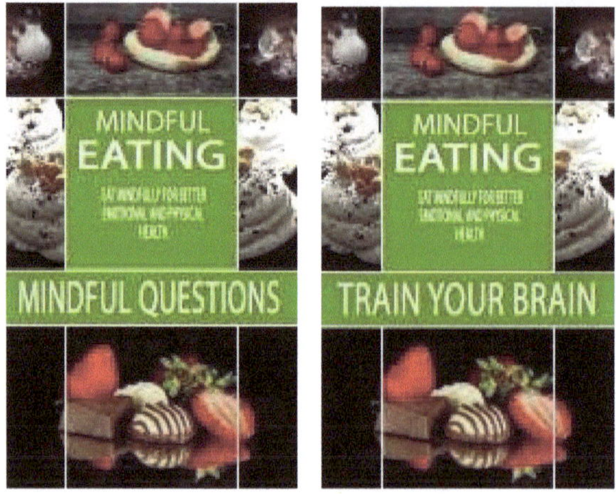

About the Author

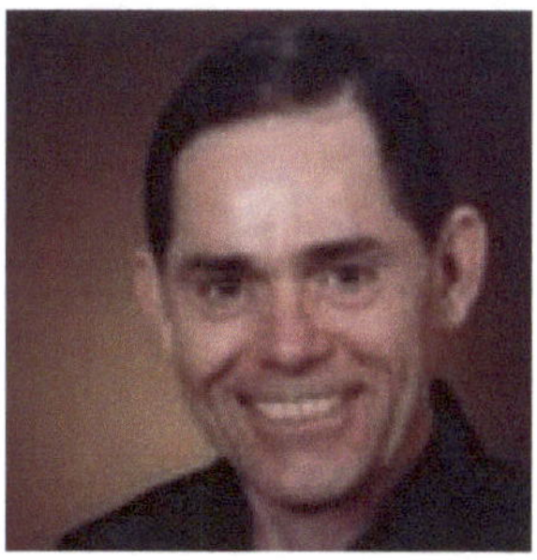

I have published over 125 books on Amazon for Kindle, CreateSpace and other publishing platforms.

While most of my books are on health and fitness in general, as I age (now 65) at the time of this writing) my topics of interest are geared toward aging baby boomers and older.

Besides my own writing, I also ghostwrite ebooks, books, reports, articles, blogs and do Kindle conversions for clients on a variety of topics.

Today my wife and I are retired from our careers and live in Gold Canyon, AZ. I now write as a retirement business where you'll find me happily sitting in my office typing away on my laptop as I work on my next book or ghostwriting project . . . that is if we are not traveling on a cruise ship - our new-found mode of travel.

9 781975 988937